EFT Tapping for Anxiety

Your 21-Day Journey to Reducing Stress

EFT Tapping with Angel

Angel Ashbrook

Anxiety.

Your heart races before a big event, or maybe just because it's Tuesday. You lie awake at 3 AM with thoughts spinning about tomorrow's to-do list.

The sight of your inbox sends you into a spiral of overwhelm. Sound familiar?

What anxiety feels like to me:

- Tight chest and shallow breathing
- Racing thoughts that won't quiet down
- Stomach in knots before social events
- Constant worry about "what if" scenarios
- Physical tension and restlessness

And here's where EFT can help with all of these. EFT (Emotional Freedom Technique) works like emotional acupuncture - but instead of needles, we use our fingertips.

By tapping specific points on your body while acknowledging your feelings, you can calm your nervous system and release anxiety within minutes.

Have you ever noticed how you instinctively rub your forehead when stressed or touch your heart when moved? Your body naturally knows where to send a soothing touch. EFT Tapping harnesses this innate wisdom, combining gentle touch with emotional release.

Why It Works:

- Tapping soothes your amygdala, the brain's stress center
- Physical touch releases calming hormones
- Speaking your truth while tapping helps process emotions
- The rhythm of tapping naturally calms your system

The Basic Process Is Simple:

1. Notice what's bothering you
2. Rate your distress level (0-10)
3. Tap through the points while expressing your feelings
4. Check in with your body
5. Rate your distress again

Think of anxiety like a tangled ball of holiday lights. Each time you tap, you untangle one more knot.

Sometimes the whole thing loosens at once; other times, you need to work with it bit by bit. Both approaches are perfectly normal and effective.

What Makes EFT Different:

- Works quickly (often in minutes)
- Can be done anywhere, anytime
- Requires no special equipment
- Combines physical relief with emotional release
- Gets to the root cause while soothing symptoms

In this book, you'll learn proven tapping sequences that target different types of anxiety.

Each script is designed to guide you through the exact words and points to use, taking the guesswork out of your healing journey.

Remember: You don't have to "believe" in EFT (yet) for it to work. You just need to follow the sequences and stay open to the possibility of feeling better.

I was skeptical at first, too (more about that in a moment). But when I saw how helpful it was in *many* areas of my life, I became an EFT practitioner myself!

And I never looked back (except to dig into my childhood trauma and work through it with EFT tapping, of course).

Chapter 1

The Science Behind EFT: How It Works

Imagine your body's stress response as a smoke alarm. Sometimes it goes off when there's real danger (an actual fire), but often it rings when you're just making toast. Anxiety works the same way - your body's alarm system gets triggered even when there's no immediate threat.

Think about the last time you felt anxious. Maybe your heart raced, your palms got sweaty, or your thoughts started spinning. That's your body's alarm system in action. It's trying to protect you, but sometimes it's a bit too enthusiastic about its job!

Here's the fascinating part: when you tap on specific points while acknowledging your feelings, you're actually:

Calming Your Stress Center

Your brain has an "anxiety button" called the amygdala. Research shows that tapping sends a signal to this button saying "you're safe," helping to turn down your body's alarm system. It's like having a remote control for your stress response!

Changing Your Brain Chemistry

When you're anxious, your body floods with stress hormones - it's preparing you to fight or run away. That's great if you're facing a lion, not so helpful when you're trying to send an email! Tapping helps:

- Lower your stress hormones
- Release natural feel-good chemicals
- Bring your heart rate back to normal
- Help you breathe more easily

Rewiring Your Response

Every time you tap while feeling anxious, you're teaching your brain a new response:

- Old pattern: Trigger → Panic → More Panic
- New pattern: Trigger → Tap → Calm

It's like creating a new path through tall grass - the more you walk it, the clearer the path becomes.

Research shows that people experience significant relief from:

- Public speaking anxiety
- Test and performance stress
- Social worries
- Work-related tension
- Health concerns
- General overwhelm

The Beautiful Truth About EFT:

- It works quickly (often within minutes)
- You can do it anywhere (even in the bathroom at work!)
- The effects are lasting
- You don't need any special equipment
- It's always available when you need it

Think of EFT as teaching your body a new language - the language of calm.

At first, it might feel a bit awkward, like learning any new skill. But soon, your body and brain start to understand that **tapping = safety**, and *that's when the magic happens*.

Chapter 2

My First Experience With Tapping

I didn't like EFT tapping at first.

When I discovered it, I was drawn to the science behind it and the potential for relief. But as someone living with anxiety every day for decades, something about the traditional approach felt "off" to me.

The standard EFT statements - ones that began with *"Even though I have this anxiety..."* or *"Even though I'm struggling..."* - made my anxiety skyrocket! As I started working with clients, I saw the same thing happen to them.

Starting with negative statements, even when followed by positive affirmations, felt like shining a spotlight on everything that was overwhelming me. My sensitive nervous system couldn't handle it.

I almost gave up on EFT entirely, especially after practitioners told me I had to do it that way to "work through" everything.

I knew the science behind it made sense, and I had read so many success stories. I wanted to keep trying. Thankfully, I didn't give up.

So I started experimenting. What if I could keep the tapping but change the statements? What if, instead of starting with what was wrong, I began with gentle curiosity?

That's when everything changed.

I developed my own approach, starting with questions like "I wonder what peace would feel like..." and "What if relaxation could flow naturally..."

These curiosity-based statements felt safer. They created space for possibility without triggering more anxiety.

Then, in the second round of tapping, once my system felt more settled, I'd move into direct positive affirmations: "I feel peace," "Relaxation flows naturally."

Combined with journaling and meditation, this gentler approach transformed my relationship with EFT. Instead of dreading the statements, I looked forward to exploring new possibilities.

My nervous system began to trust the process because it never felt forced or overwhelming.

This is the approach you'll find throughout this book. Each sequence begins with soft curiosity before moving into positive affirmations.

It's a gentle invitation to explore what's possible, allowing your nervous system to feel safe every step of the way.

Chapter 3

Where To Tap: Your Quick-Start Guide

Think of your tapping points like buttons on a remote control - each one helps change the channel from anxiety to calm.

Don't worry about being perfect; as long as you're in the general area, you're doing it right!

Your Tapping Points (From Top to Bottom)

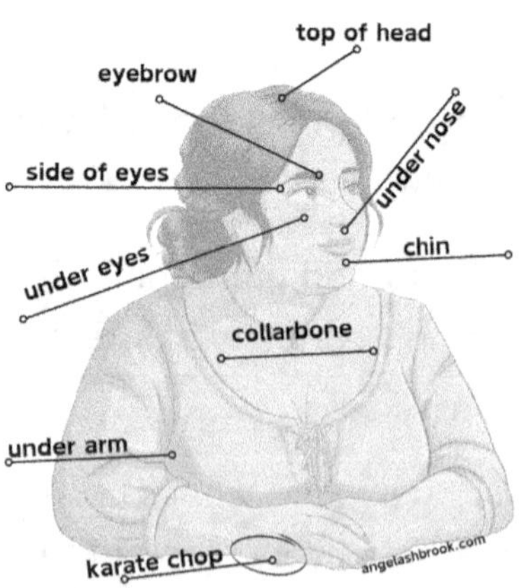

. . .

The Karate Chop Point

Find the fleshy part on the side of your hand - the spot you'd use to karate chop a board.

This is where we start. It's perfect for those moments when you're sitting at your desk, or even on the couch or (as a passenger) in the car.

I like tapping this point because even if you're surrounded by people, nobody will notice that you're tapping. Whereas if you're tapping the top of your head, the stares and comments you'll likely get will probably heighten your anxiety, not help it.

The Top of Your Head

Tap right on the crown of your head - the spot where a halo would sit. This point feels especially good when you have that tension headache from overthinking and stress.

The Eyebrow Point

Find the beginning of your eyebrow, near your nose. This is your go-to spot when you feel that familiar forehead crinkle of worry starting.

Side of Eye

Tap on the bone beside your eye - about where your smile lines might be if you were grinning. Great for when your eyes are tired from staring at your inbox too long!

Under Eye

Right on the bone under your eye, about where you'd place concealer. This point is perfect for those "I can't sleep because my mind won't shut up" moments.

Under Nose

That little groove between your nose and upper lip. (Don't worry if you're in public - you can pretend you're just thinking deeply!)

Chin Point

Find the crease between your lower lip and chin. This point is fantastic for when you're trying not to cry in frustrating situations.

Collarbone Points

Find the indent at the base of your throat, then go down about an inch and out to each side. These points are like magic buttons for chest tightness from anxiety.

Under Arm

About 4 inches below your armpit - right where your bra strap would sit. Perfect for tapping when you're alone or at home.

How to Tap

Use two fingers, or all four when it's comfortable (like on the karate chop point and collarbone)

Tap about 5-7 times on each point, but don't worry about counting or being exact - your body knows what it needs.

Pressure is like drumming your fingers on a desk - firm but gentle. Tapping should not hurt.

You can tap on either side of your body - or both if you want. I usually tap on both.

No one has ever tapped "wrong" - if you're touching the general area, it works

Feel free to tap harder or softer based on what feels good to you

Missing a point isn't a big deal - this isn't a test!

Chapter 4

How To Use This 21-Day Journey

Welcome to your pathway to peace. I've designed this book to meet you *exactly where you are*, inviting you to explore new possibilities for calm and ease in your life.

Your Daily Practice

Think of these next 21 days as gentle stepping stones. Each day offers a new opportunity to discover what peace feels like in your body, your mind, and your heart.

Morning Pages

Each day begins with a short reflection that invites you to connect with what's possible. You might be surprised at how naturally peace begins to flow when you give yourself this space.

Tapping Sequence

Following the reflection, you'll find a complete tapping sequence that gently guides you into a state of greater ease.

These sequences build upon each other, creating deeper levels of peace with each passing day.

Evening Check-In

A brief moment to notice what's shifted, what feels different, what new possibilities are opening up for you.

Remember:

- There's no "right" way to feel as you move through these practices
- You're welcome to return to any sequence that particularly resonates with you
- Feel free to adjust the words to match your own experience
- Trust that your body knows exactly what it needs

A Gentle Note About Timing

While this is structured as a 21-day journey, you're invited to move at whatever pace feels right for you.

Some days you might want to linger with a particular sequence, really allowing its medicine to sink in. Other days you might feel called to move forward.

Trust your intuition - it will guide you perfectly.

Chapter 5

Getting Started: Your First Tapping Sequence

Before we dive into our 21-day journey, let's explore a simple but powerful tapping sequence together.

Find a quiet moment where you can be present with yourself. If it feels comfortable, you might want to close your eyes.

Opening Centering Sequence

Take a soft breath in, and as you exhale, place your hand gently on your heart.

Start at the Karate Chop Point (side of your hand)

Tap gently while saying this aloud:
"I wonder what it would feel like to be completely at peace..."
"I'm open to discovering new levels of calm..."
"Relaxation flows through my body naturally..."

Round 1

Top of Head: "I invite a sense of ease..."
Eyebrow Point: "I feel safe in my body..."
Side of Eye: "I allow myself to explore these new feelings..."
Under Eye: "My body remembers how to feel calm..."
Under Nose: "Peace feels natural and easy..."
Chin: "I welcome these new possibilities..."
Collarbone: "I appreciate my body's wisdom..."
Under Arm: "I'm discovering what true calm feels like..."

Round 2

Top of Head: "Peace is already within me..."
Eyebrow Point: "I'm curious about how relaxation feels..."
Side of Eye: "Each breath brings me closer to peace..."
Under Eye: "I'm learning to trust my own wisdom..."
Under Nose: "I'm open to feeling more centered..."
Chin: "My nervous system knows how to find balance..."
Collarbone: "Each tapping point brings more peace..."
Under Arm: "Peace flows through me naturally..."

Take a gentle breath and notice what you feel in your body. What's different? What possibilities are opening up?

You can return to this sequence anytime you need a moment of centering. It's simple yet profound in its ability to shift your energy from anxiety to peace.

Chapter 6

Day 1: First Aid Anxiety Relief

Welcome to the first day of the rest of your life. Sounds cheesy, I know, but EFT Tapping truly has changed my life - and the lives of so many others. I have faith it can help change yours, too.

I remember the first time I discovered EFT. I was at my desk, completely overwhelmed by who knows what.

As someone who lived with constant anxiety, it wasn't any particular event that triggered it - anxiety was just my constant companion.

My hands were shaking, and my breath felt shallow. While I had read and watched videos about EFT tapping, I had never tried it during a panic attack.

In that moment of "what's the worst that could happen?" I began tapping, and something remarkable happened.

With each gentle tap, it felt as though someone was turning down the volume on my anxiety. Not forcing it away, but simply allowing my nervous system to remember its natural state of calm.

Like watching waves gradually smooth the sand on a beach, I felt my body settling into a more peaceful rhythm.

That's when I knew - **this simple practice could change everything.**

Since that day, EFT has become my go-to tool not just for anxiety, but for pain management, mental health, and my daily morning meditation practice. It's simple, yet profound in its ability to create real change.

Today we'll explore a powerful sequence that can bring immediate relief when anxiety feels present. Think of this as a gentle hand on your shoulder reminding you that peace is possible.

Don't get discouraged if you don't feel relief right away; everyone moves on their own timeline. Be patient and just keep tapping.

Inviting Immediate Peace

Find a comfortable space where you can be present with yourself. If it feels right, place one hand gently on your heart. Take a soft breath in... and out... allowing your body to settle.

I like to do the karate chop point to start and to end my

sequence. So, for example, karate chop point with 1-3 statements (your choice) to get you in a relaxed state.

Then all points for Round 1, all points for Round 2, and back to karate chop points to close it out.

There's no right or wrong way to do this; it's about what you feel comfortable with.

Karate Chop Point

"I wonder what it would feel like to be completely at peace..."
"I'm curious about what calm feels like in my body..."
"Relaxation flows naturally through me..."

Round 1

Eyebrow Point: "I welcome this moment of connection..."
Side of Eye: "Each breath brings me closer to center..."
Under Eye: "My nervous system knows how to find balance..."
Under Nose: "Calm feels natural and easy..."
Chin: "My body is learning this new way..."
Collarbone: "I appreciate my body's wisdom..."
Under Arm: "I'm discovering my own path to calm..."
Top of Head: "I invite spaciousness into my mind..."

Round 2

Eyebrow Point: "My body remembers how to feel calm..."
Side of Eye: "I'm discovering what peace feels like..."
Under Eye: "I allow my shoulders to soften..."
Under Nose: "I'm open to experiencing deep peace..."
Chin: "Each tap brings more ease..."
Collarbone: "Peace flows through me naturally..."
Under Arm: "Each moment brings new possibilities..."
Top of Head: "Peace is already within me..."

Take a gentle breath and notice:

- Where do you feel more spacious?
- What has shifted in your body?
- What new sensations are you discovering?

Quick Emergency Version

When you need immediate relief, focus on these key points while breathing deeply:

1. Collarbone points: "Peace is possible..."
2. Side of eye: "My body knows how to calm..."
3. Under nose: "I welcome ease..."

Evening Reflection: Take a moment to notice three moments today where you felt even slightly more peaceful. What made those moments possible?

Chapter 7

Day 2: Morning Anxiety Release

Mornings can often feel particularly challenging when anxiety is present. Today we'll explore how to start your day from a place of peaceful possibility rather than rushing anxiety.

You know those mornings - the alarm sounds and before your feet even touch the floor, your mind is already racing with everything you need to do.

The weight of the day ahead feels heavy before it's even begun. I used to dread mornings, lying in bed trying to gather the courage to face another anxious day.

But this morning sequence changed everything for me. Now it's the foundation of my daily practice, setting a tone of peace that carries through my entire day.

Creating a Peaceful Morning

Before we begin, take a soft breath and notice the gentle rhythm of your heart. If it feels comfortable, place your hand there, feeling its steady presence.

Karate Chop Point

"I wonder what it would feel like to wake up peaceful..."
"I'm open to experiencing a calm morning..."
"This day is unfolding with grace..."

Round 1

Eyebrow Point: "I welcome this moment of connection..."
Side of Eye: "Each breath brings me closer to center..."
Under Eye: "My nervous system knows how to find balance..."
Under Nose: "Calm feels natural and easy..."
Chin: "My body is learning this new way..."
Collarbone: "I appreciate my body's wisdom..."
Under Arm: "I'm discovering my own path to calm..."
Top of Head: "I invite spaciousness into my mind..."

Round 2

Eyebrow Point: "My body remembers how to feel calm..."
Side of Eye: "I'm discovering what peace feels like..."
Under Eye: "I allow my shoulders to soften..."
Under Nose: "I'm open to experiencing deep peace..."
Chin: "Each tap brings more ease..."
Collarbone: "Peace flows through me naturally..."
Under Arm: "Each moment brings new possibilities..."
Top of Head: "Peace is already within me..."

Take a gentle breath and notice:

- How has your breathing shifted?
- Where do you feel more spacious?
- What possibilities are opening up for your day?

Quick Emergency Version (for rushed mornings)

Focus on these points while taking slow breaths:

1. Top of head: "I choose peace..."
2. Collarbone: "I have enough time..."
3. Under eye: "I move with grace..."

Evening Reflection: Notice how today's morning differed from usual. What small shifts made space for more peace? What would you like to invite in tomorrow morning?

Chapter 8

Day 3: Physical Symptoms Of Anxiety

Today, I'd like for us to explore how to bring peace to those physical sensations that often accompany anxiety - the racing heart, tight chest, butterfly stomach, or tense shoulders.

Let's discover how your body can shift from tension to ease.

Most of my clients (and I) started our anxiety healing journey here - with the physical symptoms. You might not be able to control your thoughts yet, but you can feel your racing heart or tight shoulders.

These physical sensations often feel like unwelcome visitors in our body, creating even more anxiety as we notice them.

When I first started using EFT, I was amazed at how quickly the physical symptoms began to shift. My shoulders would soften, my breathing would deepen, and that knot in my stomach would begin to unwind.

It's important to remember that we're not trying to force these sensations away. Instead, you're inviting your body to remember its natural state of calm. Your body knows exactly how to relax; sometimes it just needs a gentle reminder.

Soothing Physical Tension

Gently place one hand where you most often feel anxiety in your body. Take a soft breath, allowing your hand to rise and fall with each breath. Notice how your body responds to this simple act of self-connection.

Karate Chop Point

"I wonder what complete physical ease feels like…"

"I'm curious about how relaxation flows through my body…"

"My body remembers its natural state…"

Round 1

Eyebrow Point: "I welcome relief into my shoulders…"

Side of Eye: "My heart can find its peaceful rhythm…"

Under Eye: "I'm discovering what relaxation feels like…"

Under Nose: "I allow my chest to soften and expand…"

Chin: "My muscles remember how to relax…"

Collarbone: "My nervous system is learning to reset…"

Under Arm: "I'm creating new patterns of ease…"

Top of Head: "I invite softness into every cell…"

Round 2

Eyebrow Point: "Tension melts away naturally..."

Side of Eye: "Each breath brings more ease..."

Under Eye: "My stomach can feel peaceful and calm..."

Under Nose: "Each exhale releases more tension..."

Chin: "I welcome this wave of peace..."

Collarbone: "Peace flows through my entire body..."

Under Arm: "My body thanks me for this moment..."

Top of Head: "My body knows how to find balance..."

Take a gentle breath and notice:

- Where do you feel more spacious?
- What sensations have shifted?
- Where is your body feeling more at ease?

Quick Emergency Version (for intense physical symptoms)

Focus on these points while breathing deeply:

1. Karate chop: "My body knows how to calm..."
2. Under eye: "I welcome deep peace..."
3. Collarbone: "Each breath brings relief..."

Evening Reflection: Notice the moments today when your body felt more at ease. What helped create those peaceful moments? How did your body thank you for this attention?

Chapter 9
Day 4: Racing Thoughts

Today we'll explore how to bring spaciousness to a mind that feels busy with thoughts. Let's discover how your mind can shift from racing to peaceful clarity.

Racing thoughts were always there, no matter how well my day was going.

You know that feeling when your mind seems to be running a marathon even while you're sitting still? One thought chasing the next, spinning stories about what might happen, replaying conversations that already did.

EFT was a revelation because it gave me a way to create space between these thoughts, like opening windows in a stuffy room.

Your mind's natural state is clarity. Just as clouds pass through the sky without changing its vast nature, thoughts can move through your mind without disturbing your inner peace.

We're not trying to empty your mind, we just want to create a bit more breathing room between thoughts.

Finding Mental Clarity

Find a comfortable position and, if you'd like, close your eyes. Take a gentle breath and imagine your thoughts like clouds in a vast sky - there's so much space around them.

Karate Chop Point

"I wonder what mental spaciousness feels like..."

"I'm open to discovering clarity beneath these thoughts..."

"What if peace could flow through my mind naturally..."

Round 1

Eyebrow Point: "I welcome moments of mental clarity..."

Side of Eye: "I allow my mind to settle..."

Under Eye: "I'm discovering what mental peace feels like..."

Under Nose: "I welcome this moment of quiet..."

Chin: "My mind remembers how to be still..."

Collarbone: "My thoughts can settle like snow in a globe..."

Under Arm: "I'm creating new patterns of mental ease..."

Top of Head: "I invite stillness into my thoughts..."

Round 2

Eyebrow Point: "What if these thoughts could slow naturally..."

Side of Eye: "Each breath brings more space..."

Under Eye: "My thoughts can flow with ease..."

Under Nose: "Each exhale creates more space..."

Chin: "I appreciate these moments of clarity..."

Collarbone: "Peace flows through my mind..."

Under Arm: "Each moment brings more clarity..."

Top of Head: "My mind knows how to find quiet..."

Take a gentle breath and notice:

- Where do you feel more spacious in your mind?
- What has shifted in your thought patterns?
- What new sense of peace are you discovering?

Quick Emergency Version (for overwhelming thought moments)

Focus on these points while taking slow breaths:

1. Top of head: "I allow my mind to settle..."
2. Karate Chop Point: "I welcome clarity..."
3. Sides of eyes: "Peace flows naturally..."

Evening Reflection: Notice the moments today when your mind felt clearer. What created those peaceful spaces? How did it feel to experience those moments of mental quiet?

Chapter 10
Day 5: Future Worries

The future can feel like a movie playing in our minds - endless scenes of "what if" and "what might be."

I've spent decades living five steps ahead, my mind constantly spinning stories about tomorrow while missing the peace available today. That's why this sequence became one of my daily anchors.

When we're caught up in future worries, our bodies often forget we're safe right now. Our shoulders tense, our breathing shallows, and we lose connection with the present moment. EFT gives us a way to gently return to now, where peace is always waiting.

Finding Peace with the Future

Take a gentle breath and place your feet firmly on the ground. Feel the support beneath you, right here in this moment. Let your shoulders soften as you connect with the present.

Karate Chop Point
"I choose to trust in my future..."
"I am open to peaceful possibilities..."
"Each step forward feels secure and clear..."

Round 1

Eyebrow Point: "My path is becoming clearer..."
Side of Eye: "I am grounded and centered..."
Under Eye: "Trust flows naturally through me..."
Under Nose: "I am present and peaceful..."
Chin: "My future self is peaceful and wise..."
Collarbone: "The present moment nourishes me..."
Under Arm: "I create my future from peace..."
Top of Head: "I trust in divine timing..."

Round 2

Eyebrow Point: "Everything is working out wonderfully..."
Side of Eye: "This moment holds wisdom..."
Under Eye: "My path is unfolding with grace..."
Under Nose: "Each breath centers me in now..."
Chin: "Divine timing guides my path..."
Collarbone: "Peace flows through every moment..."
Under Arm: "Each step forward brings clarity..."
Top of Head: "Each day unfolds perfectly..."

Take a gentle breath and notice:

- Where do you feel most grounded?
- How has your relationship with the future shifted?
- What new sense of trust is emerging?

Quick Emergency Version (for future worry spirals)

Focus on these points while taking slow breaths:

1. Collarbone: "I am safe right now"
2. Under eye: "Divine timing guides me"
3. Top of head: "All is well"

Evening Reflection: Notice the moments today when you felt at peace with what lies ahead. What helped you find that trust? How did it feel to rest in the present moment?

Chapter 11

Day 6: Social Anxiety

Walking into a room full of people used to feel like stepping onto a stage without knowing my lines. My heart would race, my palms would sweat, and my mind would flood with worries about what others might think.

Social anxiety isn't just about being shy - it's about our nervous system going into overdrive in social situations. Now I'm not saying I'm magically cured because I use EFT tapping, but I do have the tools to calm myself down even in tough situations (like being surrounded by people who expect me to have something to say).

What I love about EFT tapping for social anxiety is that we can tap anywhere, anytime. Standing in line at a coffee shop, sitting in your car before a meeting, or even in a bathroom stall at a party - these moments of tapping can help your system remember that you're safe, capable, and worthy of connection just as you are.

Finding Peace in Social Spaces

Take a gentle breath and feel the space around you. Notice how this space already holds you with acceptance. Let your body soften as you connect with your own natural presence.

Karate Chop Point
"I move through social spaces with ease..."
"I am naturally magnetic..."
"My presence brings value to every interaction..."

Round 1

Eyebrow Point: "I connect effortlessly with others..."
Side of Eye: "I am at ease in every gathering..."
Under Eye: "Joy flows naturally in my interactions..."
Under Nose: "I am perfectly myself in all situations..."
Chin: "I speak my truth with grace..."
Collarbone: "I belong in every space I enter..."
Under Arm: "I create warmth wherever I go..."
Top of Head: "I radiate peaceful confidence..."

Round 2

Eyebrow Point: "My words flow naturally and clearly..."
Side of Eye: "My energy is warm and inviting..."
Under Eye: "I bring light to every conversation..."
Under Nose: "My presence is a gift..."
Chin: "Connection flows easily through me..."
Collarbone: "Peace fills all my interactions..."
Under Arm: "My social energy flows naturally..."
Top of Head: "My authentic self shines brightly..."

Take a gentle breath and notice:

- Where do you feel most connected to yourself?
- How has your sense of presence shifted?
- What new feeling of ease is emerging?

Quick Emergency Version (for social situations)

Focus on these points while taking slow breaths:

1. Collarbone: "I am naturally at ease"
2. Under eye: "I connect authentically"
3. Top of head: "My presence is enough"

If you're surrounded by people, you can tap the karate chop point without anyone noticing. Do that, while saying these statements in your head and taking slow, calming breaths.

Evening Reflection: Notice the moments today when social connections felt easy and natural. What helped you find that flow? How did it feel to share your authentic presence?

Chapter 12

Day 7: Self-Trust Building

Have you ever noticed how anxiety makes us doubt our own inner knowing? For years, I second-guessed every decision, seeking validation from everyone except myself.

The constant questioning was exhausting. But beneath all that noise, our inner wisdom is always waiting - calm, clear, and surprisingly trustworthy.

What I love most about tapping for self-trust is how it creates space to simply listen to ourselves.

Not the anxious chatter of "what-ifs," but that quiet, steady voice that knows exactly what we need.

As we tap, that voice grows stronger, and trusting ourselves becomes as natural as breathing.

Deepening Self-Trust

Take a gentle breath and place your hand on your heart. Feel the wisdom that already lives in your body. Let yourself settle into this knowing presence within you.

Karate Chop Point
"I trust my inner guidance completely..."
"My wisdom flows naturally..."
"Every decision I make is perfect for me..."

Round 1

Eyebrow Point: "I listen to my inner voice with ease..."
Side of Eye: "I trust my path completely..."
Under Eye: "Wisdom flows naturally through me..."
Under Nose: "I am my own best guide..."
Chin: "I move forward with certainty..."
Collarbone: "I trust myself deeply..."
Under Arm: "My decisions bring peace..."
Top of Head: "My intuition guides me clearly..."

Round 2

Eyebrow Point: "My choices align with my highest good..."
Side of Eye: "My decisions create beautiful outcomes..."
Under Eye: "I follow my heart with confidence..."
Under Nose: "My inner knowing speaks clearly..."
Chin: "Every choice reveals more wisdom..."
Collarbone: "My path unfolds perfectly..."
Under Arm: "Self-trust flows naturally through me..."
Top of Head: "I know exactly what I need..."

Take a gentle breath and notice:

- Where do you feel this natural wisdom in your body?
- How has your connection to your intuition deepened?
- What new sense of certainty is emerging?

Quick Emergency Version (for decision moments)

Focus on these points while taking slow breaths:

1. Collarbone: "I trust myself completely"
2. Under eye: "My wisdom› guides me perfectly"
3. Top of head: "I know my truth"

Evening Reflection: Notice the moments today when you felt deeply connected to your inner wisdom. What helped you find that trust? How did it feel to move through your day with complete self-trust?

Quick Note from Angel

Amazing work reaching this point in your EFT tapping journey! Have you been following along with my YouTube videos?

The neural pathways you're building through consistent tapping practice are getting stronger each day.

Habits start getting easier to stick with around day 7-8 - right where you are now.

Take a moment to notice what's shifted since you began:

- How does your body respond differently to stress?
- What anxious moments feel more manageable?
- Where do you notice more natural calm?

Even if the changes feel subtle, *they're significant.* Your nervous system is learning a new way of being. Just keep tapping!

Chapter 13

Day 8: Past Anxiety Experiences

Sometimes our nervous system gets stuck in old stories, replaying past moments of anxiety as if they're happening right now.

I know this pattern well - certain memories would trigger my anxiety response even years later. But those same experiences that once felt overwhelming can become stepping stones to deeper wisdom.

EFT offers a gentle way to revisit these memories while staying anchored in present safety.

It's like watching old home movies from a comfortable distance - we can acknowledge what happened while knowing we're different now, stronger now, wiser now.

Transforming Past Experiences

Take a gentle breath and feel the ground beneath you. Notice how this present moment holds you securely. Let your body settle into the safety of now.

Karate Chop Point
"I embrace all my experiences as wisdom..."
"I grow stronger every day..."
"My past guides me toward peace..."

Round 1

Eyebrow Point: "I transform every memory into wisdom..."
Side of Eye: "I see my journey with compassion..."
Under Eye: "Peace flows through all my memories..."
Under Nose: "I am exactly where I need to be..."
Chin: "My experiences shape my strength..."
Collarbone: "I learn and grow naturally..."
Under Arm: "My past creates beautiful wisdom..."
Top of Head: "I am safe in this moment..."

Round 2

Eyebrow Point: "My experiences make me stronger..."
Side of Eye: "Each step leads to greater peace..."
Under Eye: "I embrace my whole story..."
Under Nose: "My path unfolds perfectly..."
Chin: "I welcome all parts of my journey..."
Collarbone: "Every moment brings new understanding..."
Under Arm: "I move forward with grace..."
Top of Head: "Every experience brings growth..."

Take a gentle breath and notice:

- Where do you feel this new strength in your body?
- How has your relationship with your past shifted?
- What new understanding is emerging?

Quick Emergency Version (for triggered moments)

Focus on these points while taking slow breaths:

1. Collarbone: "I am safe now"
2. Under eye: "I transform every experience"
3. Top of head: "Peace flows through my story"

Evening Reflection: Notice the moments today when past experiences felt lighter. What helped you find that transformation? How did it feel to embrace your journey with compassion?

Chapter 14
Day 9: Work/School Stress

The endless to-do list. The looming deadlines. The pressure to perform perfectly. Work, school, and life in general can feel like pressure cookers for anxiety, turning even tasks we enjoy into sources of stress.

I discovered EFT during a particularly overwhelming work period, and it changed everything about how I approach my professional life.

The beauty of tapping for work stress is that we can shift from pushing ourselves harder to allowing our natural capabilities to shine through.

When we're not fighting anxiety, we often find we're far more capable than we imagined. Our mind clears, our focus sharpens, and productivity becomes a natural flow rather than a forced march.

Finding Peace in Performance

Take a gentle breath and straighten your spine gently. Feel the natural dignity in your posture. Let your shoulders relax as you connect with your innate capabilities.

Karate Chop Point
"I accomplish tasks with ease..."
"My mind works clearly and efficiently..."
"Success flows naturally through me..."

Round 1

Eyebrow Point: "I focus naturally and easily..."
Side of Eye: "I manage my time perfectly..."
Under Eye: "Ideas flow effortlessly to me..."
Under Nose: "I contribute valuable work..."
Chin: "I balance my energy perfectly..."
Collarbone: "I accomplish goals with ease..."
Under Arm: "I create outstanding results..."
Top of Head: "I handle every task brilliantly..."

Round 2

Eyebrow Point: "My work brings satisfaction..."
Side of Eye: "Every project unfolds smoothly..."
Under Eye: "I complete everything with grace..."
Under Nose: "My efforts bring excellent results..."
Chin: "My productivity flows naturally..."
Collarbone: "Success comes naturally to me..."
Under Arm: "My work energizes me..."
Top of Head: "My energy supports my success..."

Take a gentle breath and notice:

- Where do you feel this natural confidence?
- How has your relationship with work shifted?
- What new sense of capability is emerging?

Quick Emergency Version (for deadline pressure)

Focus on these points while taking slow breaths:

1. Collarbone: "I work with natural flow"
2. Under eye: "Everything completes perfectly"
3. Top of head: "I create excellent results"

Evening Reflection: Notice the moments today when work felt effortless. What helped you find that flow? How did it feel to move through tasks with natural confidence?

Chapter 15

Day 10: Family Tensions

Family relationships can be some of our deepest sources of both joy and anxiety. Those old patterns, unspoken expectations, and complicated dynamics often trigger our nervous system in ways that other relationships don't.

I discovered that when I could stay peaceful within myself, even challenging family moments became opportunities for deeper connection.

EFT offers a beautiful way to stay centered in family situations. Instead of getting caught in reactive patterns, we can tap into a place of calm presence.

From this space, we often find that the very dynamics that once triggered anxiety can transform into pathways for growth and understanding.

Creating Family Harmony

Take a gentle breath and feel your heart space expand. Notice how love naturally flows when you're at peace. Let your body relax into this space of acceptance.

Karate Chop Point

"I radiate peace in all interactions..."
"Love flows easily through me..."
"I create harmony naturally..."

Round 1

Eyebrow Point: "I see beyond surface tensions..."
Side of Eye: "I communicate with clarity..."
Under Eye: "Peace flows through all relationships..."
Under Nose: "I remain centered and calm..."
Chin: "I choose responses that serve peace..."
Collarbone: "I maintain my inner peace..."
Under Arm: "I create positive connections..."
Top of Head: "I respond with wisdom..."

Round 2

Eyebrow Point: "Understanding flows naturally..."
Side of Eye: "My words create connection..."
Under Eye: "I bring light to every interaction..."
Under Nose: "My boundaries create harmony..."
Chin: "My heart stays open and clear..."
Collarbone: "Love guides all my actions..."
Under Arm: "Harmony flows through my family..."
Top of Head: "My presence brings calm..."

Take a gentle breath and notice:

- Where do you feel this natural harmony?
- How has your approach to relationships shifted?
- What new sense of peace is emerging?

Quick Emergency Version (for tense moments)

Focus on these points while taking slow breaths:

1. Collarbone: "I remain peaceful"
2. Under eye: "I respond with love"
3. Top of head: "Harmony flows naturally"

Evening Reflection: Notice the moments today when family interactions felt peaceful. What helped you find that harmony? How did it feel to maintain your center while connecting with others?

Chapter 16

Day 11: Health Anxiety

Every sensation in our body can become a source of worry when health anxiety is present.

A simple headache turns into catastrophic thoughts, a random pain spawns endless Google searches. I lived this way for years, until EFT helped me discover a new way of listening to my body - not with fear, but with understanding.

What makes tapping so powerful for health anxiety is that it helps us strengthen our relationship with our body's innate wisdom.

Instead of fighting against every sensation, we can create a gentle dialogue with our body, trusting that it knows how to maintain balance and heal.

Embracing Wellness

Take a gentle breath and feel the living energy in your body.

Notice how your body supports you in every moment. Let yourself settle into this natural vitality.

Karate Chop Point
"My body knows perfect health..."
"Wellness flows through me..."
"I trust my body's wisdom..."

Round 1

Eyebrow Point: "I listen to my body with love..."
Side of Eye: "I trust my body completely..."
Under Eye: "My body maintains perfect balance..."
Under Nose: "I embrace vibrant wellness..."
Chin: "I support my natural health..."
Collarbone: "My body restores itself naturally..."
Under Arm: "I create perfect wellness..."
Top of Head: "My body functions perfectly..."

Round 2

Eyebrow Point: "My healing abilities work naturally..."
Side of Eye: "Wellness comes easily to me..."
Under Eye: "Health flows through every cell..."
Under Nose: "My body knows exactly what it needs..."
Chin: "My immune system works perfectly..."
Collarbone: "I maintain radiant health..."
Under Arm: "My body thrives naturally..."
Top of Head: "Health radiates through me..."

Take a gentle breath and notice:

- Where do you feel this natural vitality?
- How has your connection to your body shifted?
- What new sense of wellness is emerging?

Quick Emergency Version (for health concern moments)

Focus on these points while taking slow breaths:

1. Collarbone: "My body knows health"
2. Under eye: "I trust my healing"
3. Top of head: "Wellness flows naturally"

Evening Reflection: Notice the moments today when you felt connected to your body's wisdom. What helped you find that trust? How did it feel to embrace your natural wellness?

Chapter 17

Day 12: Financial Worries

Money worries can create some of the most persistent anxiety patterns, affecting our sleep, relationships, and daily peace of mind.

I understand this deeply - it's why I created an entire book on EFT Tapping for financial freedom.

This sequence offers a gentle introduction to transforming your relationship with money.

Financial anxiety often shows up as a tightness in our chest or a knot in our stomach every time we check our bank account or open a bill.

Through tapping, we can begin to release these physical tension patterns, allowing our nervous system to settle into a state where clearer financial decisions become possible.

Creating Financial Peace

Take a gentle breath and feel the abundance that already exists around you. Notice the resources that support you in every moment. Let your body relax into this natural flow.

Karate Chop Point
"Money flows easily to me..."
"I attract abundance naturally..."
"Prosperity surrounds me..."

Round 1

Eyebrow Point: "I manage money wisely..."
Side of Eye: "I trust in divine supply..."
Under Eye: "Money works for me..."
Under Nose: "I attract opportunities easily..."
Chin: "I deserve financial success..."
Collarbone: "I enjoy financial freedom..."
Under Arm: "I create lasting wealth..."
Top of Head: "I create wealth easily..."

Round 2

Eyebrow Point: "Financial success comes naturally..."
Side of Eye: "My income grows steadily..."
Under Eye: "Abundance flows in perfect timing..."
Under Nose: "My wealth expands naturally..."
Chin: "Money comes to me in expected and unexpected ways..." **Collarbone:** "Abundance supports me perfectly..."
Under Arm: "Money flows naturally in my life..."
Top of Head: "Abundance fills my life..."

Take a gentle breath and notice:

- Where do you feel this natural abundance?
- How has your relationship with money shifted?
- What new sense of prosperity is emerging?

Quick Emergency Version (for money worry moments)

Focus on these points while taking slow breaths:

1. Collarbone: "I trust in abundance"
2. Under eye: "Money flows easily"
3. Top of head: "I am financially secure"

Evening Reflection: Notice the moments today when you felt financially peaceful. What helped you find that trust? How did it feel to embrace your natural abundance?

Chapter 18

Day 13: Performance Anxiety

Whether it's a work presentation, an audition, or speaking at an event, performance anxiety can transform exciting opportunities into moments of dread.

The racing heart, shaky voice, sweaty palms - I know these feelings intimately. EFT became my secret weapon before presentations, allowing me to channel that nervous energy into authentic presence.

The amazing thing about tapping for performance anxiety is how it helps us access the natural confidence that's always within us. Instead of trying to suppress our nerves, we create space for both excitement and calm to coexist.

When we're not fighting our anxiety, our true talents can shine through effortlessly.

Embracing Your Spotlight

Take a gentle breath and feel your natural presence. Notice the power that already lives within you. Let your body settle into your confidence.

Karate Chop Point
"I shine naturally in every moment..."
"My presence captivates..."
"I perform with effortless grace..."

Round 1

Eyebrow Point: "I communicate with clarity..."
Side of Eye: "I embrace every opportunity..."
Under Eye: "I connect authentically with my audience..."
Under Nose: "I share my gifts easily..."
Chin: "I embody natural confidence..."
Collarbone: "I inspire others naturally..."
Under Arm: "I create magical moments..."
Top of Head: "I express myself perfectly..."

Round 2

Eyebrow Point: "My message lands powerfully..."
Side of Eye: "My performance flows naturally..."
Under Eye: "My presence engages naturally..."
Under Nose: "My voice carries strength..."
Chin: "My excellence shines through..."
Collarbone: "My performance uplifts..."
Under Arm: "Success flows through my performance..."
Top of Head: "My talents flow freely..."

Take a gentle breath and notice:

- Where do you feel this natural confidence?
- How has your relationship with performance shifted?
- What new sense of ease is emerging?

Quick Emergency Version (for performance moments)

Focus on these points while taking slow breaths:

1. Collarbone: "I perform naturally"
2. Under eye: "I shine effortlessly"
3. Top of head: "I engage perfectly"

Evening Reflection: Notice the moments today when you felt confident in the spotlight. What helped you find that flow? How did it feel to share your gifts naturally?

Chapter 19
Day 14: Perfectionism

Perfectionism feels like a constant editor sitting on your shoulder, critiquing every move, every word, every decision.

For years, I felt trapped in a cycle of perfectionism without realizing it. Success brought no relief - just higher standards and harsher self-judgment.

Every achievement became another bar to clear, another chance to prove *I still wasn't doing enough*. Even when my logical mind knew these standards were impossible, my nervous system stayed locked in high alert, constantly scanning for flaws.

That's what made EFT so transformative - it gave me tools to release this pattern at the deepest level.

The irony of perfectionism is that it actually blocks our natural excellence. When we're caught in the grip of "not good enough," we can't access our creativity and wisdom.

Tapping helps us release this grip, allowing our authentic capabilities to emerge without the constant pressure of perfection.

Embracing Natural Excellence

Take a gentle breath and feel the fullness of who you are. Notice the completeness that exists in this moment. Let your body settle into this natural state of being enough.

Karate Chop Point

"I embrace my natural excellence..."
"I flow with ease..."
"My best is absolutely perfect..."

Round 1

Eyebrow Point: "I love my authentic expression..."
Side of Eye: "I create with natural flow..."
Under Eye: "I trust my natural process..."
Under Nose: "I am enough exactly as I am..."
Chin: "I celebrate my unique path..."
Collarbone: "I move forward with ease..."
Under Arm: "I create magnificent results..."
Top of Head: "I release the need to prove..."

Round 2

Eyebrow Point: "My way is exactly right..."
Side of Eye: "My efforts bring beautiful results..."
Under Eye: "Everything unfolds perfectly..."
Under Nose: "My work reflects my true self..."
Chin: "My excellence shines naturally..."
Collarbone: "Every step brings perfect growth..."
Under Arm: "My natural flow brings success..."
Top of Head: "Excellence flows naturally..."

Take a gentle breath and notice:

- Where do you feel this natural excellence?
- How has your approach to achievement shifted?
- What new sense of ease is emerging?

Quick Emergency Version (for perfectionist moments)

Focus on these points while taking slow breaths:

1. Collarbone: "I am naturally perfect"
2. Under eye: "I flow with ease"
3. Top of head: "My best is enough"

Evening Reflection: Notice the moments today when excellence flowed naturally. What helped you find that ease? How did it feel to release perfectionism and embrace your natural flow?

Chapter 20

Day 15: Decision Making Anxiety

Making decisions used to feel like walking through a maze blindfolded - every choice weighted with the fear of making the "wrong" move.

Even small decisions would keep me up at night, my mind endlessly cycling through all possible outcomes.

The beautiful thing about tapping for decision anxiety is that it helps quiet the endless "what-ifs" so we can hear our own inner knowing.

When we're not caught in anxiety's grip, we often find that we already know exactly what feels right for us. It's not about making perfect decisions - it's about trusting our ability to handle whatever outcome unfolds.

Embracing Clear Decisions

Take a gentle breath and feel your spirit's wisdom. Notice the guidance that already lives within you. Let your body settle into this natural knowing.

Karate Chop Point
"I accept the outcome of my decisions..."
"My choices create beautiful outcomes..."
"Clarity flows naturally to me..."

Round 1

Eyebrow Point: "I trust my inner guidance..."
Side of Eye: "I see my options clearly..."
Under Eye: "I move forward with confidence..."
Under Nose: "I choose naturally and easily..."
Chin: "I trust each step I take..."
Collarbone: "I decide with complete clarity..."
Under Arm: "I create positive outcomes..."
Top of Head: "I know exactly what I need..."

Round 2

Eyebrow Point: "My decisions bring positive results..."
Side of Eye: "Each choice reveals more wisdom..."
Under Eye: "My decisions align with my highest good..."
Under Nose: "My inner compass guides me perfectly..."
Chin: "My choices create success..."
Collarbone: "Every decision serves my growth..."
Under Arm: "My choices flow with ease..."
Top of Head: "My path unfolds perfectly..."

Take a gentle breath and notice:

- Where do you feel this natural clarity?
- How has your approach to decisions shifted?
- What new sense of confidence is emerging?

Quick Emergency Version (for decision moments)

Focus on these points while taking slow breaths:

1. Collarbone: "I choose clearly"
2. Under eye: "I trust my decisions"
3. Top of head: "My path is perfect"

Evening Reflection: Notice the moments today when decisions felt clear and natural. What helped you find that clarity? How did it feel to trust your choices completely?

Chapter 21

Day 16: Fear Of Change

Our bodies are wired to seek safety in the familiar, even when that familiar place isn't serving us anymore. I remember how paralyzed I felt when facing big changes - my nervous system treating every new opportunity like a threat.

EFT taught me that we can retrain this response, allowing change to feel more like an adventure than a danger.

When we tap through fear of change, we remind our nervous system that we're designed for growth and adaptation.

Just like a plant naturally turns toward the sun, we have this natural capacity to flow with life's transitions. Tapping helps us access this natural resilience beneath the fear.

Embracing Beautiful Changes

Take a gentle breath and notice how your body is already changing with each inhale and exhale. Feel how naturally you flow with these small changes. Your body knows how to adapt and grow.

Karate Chop Point

"I wonder what exciting possibilities change brings..."
"I'm open to life's natural unfolding..."
"Each change brings gifts and opportunities..."

Round 1

Eyebrow Point: "I welcome fresh perspectives..."
Side of Eye: "I see the beauty in transformation..."
Under Eye: "I trust life's natural evolution..."
Under Nose: "I embrace new beginnings..."
Chin: "I welcome this journey of growth..."
Collarbone: "I trust in divine timing..."
Under Arm: "I create beautiful transformations..."
Top of Head: "I flow easily with life's rhythm..."

Round 2

Eyebrow Point: "Each shift brings more clarity..."
Side of Eye: "Change opens doors to growth..."
Under Eye: "Each change brings perfect timing..."
Under Nose: "Change flows gracefully through me..."
Chin: "Each shift reveals more wisdom..."
Collarbone: "Change guides me to my highest good..."
Under Arm: "Each change brings more peace..."
Top of Head: "Change reveals new paths of joy..."

Take a gentle breath and notice:

- Where do you feel most open to change?
- What new possibilities are emerging?
- How has your relationship with change shifted?

Quick Emergency Version (for moments of resistance to change)

Focus on these points while taking slow breaths:

1. Collarbone: "I trust this unfolding"
2. Under eye: "Change brings gifts"
3. Top of head: "I flow with ease"

Evening Reflection: Notice the moments today when change felt natural and exciting. What helped you embrace these shifts? How did it feel to welcome transformation?

Chapter 22
Day 17: Creating Safety

Our nervous systems are brilliantly designed with a built-in safety scanner, constantly assessing our environment for threats.

In our modern world, this ancient survival mechanism can become oversensitive, perceiving danger even in safe situations.

But here's the amazing thing - through EFT, we can actually rewire these neural pathways, teaching our brain to recognize safety as easily as it spots potential threats.

This is where the science of neuroplasticity meets the wisdom of EFT. Each time we tap while focusing on safety, we're strengthening new neural connections.

We're literally training our nervous system to expand its "safe zone," allowing our bodies to recognize and settle into security more naturally.

Embodying Safety

Take a gentle breath and feel the safety that surrounds you. Notice the strength in your own body. Let yourself settle into this natural security.

Karate Chop Point
"I am completely safe..."
"Security flows through me..."
"I create safety wherever I go..."

Round 1

Eyebrow Point: "I anchor deeply in safety..."
Side of Eye: "I recognize my security..."
Under Eye: "I feel protected and secure..."
Under Nose: "I trust my surroundings..."
Chin: "I create secure spaces..."
Collarbone: "I am naturally protected..."
Under Arm: "I attract safe experiences..."
Top of Head: "I trust my environment..."

Round 2

Eyebrow Point: "My world supports me perfectly..."
Side of Eye: "Peace flows through my space..."
Under Eye: "Safety radiates from within..."
Under Nose: "My environment nurtures me..."
Chin: "Safety flows naturally to me..."
Collarbone: "Security fills my world..."
Under Arm: "Protection surrounds me always..."
Top of Head: "Safety surrounds me always..."

Take a gentle breath and notice:

- Where do you feel this natural safety?
- How has your sense of security deepened?
- What new feeling of protection is emerging?

Quick Emergency Version

Focus on these points while taking slow breaths:

1. Collarbone: "I am completely safe"
2. Under eye: "Security surrounds me"
3. Top of head: "I trust my safety"

Evening Reflection: Notice the moments today when you felt deeply secure. What helped you find that safety? How did it feel to move through your day with complete protection?

Chapter 23
Day 18: Building Confidence

Pause for a moment and celebrate - you've come so far on this journey! With just a few days remaining, notice how differently you feel from when you started.

Your commitment to this practice is creating beautiful transformations.

Research shows that confidence isn't just a mindset - it's actually a physiological state our nervous system can learn and remember.

Each time we tap while connecting to our inner strength, we're reinforcing neural pathways that make confidence feel more natural and accessible.

It's like creating a well-worn path in our brain that makes it easier to access our natural authority.

What fascinates me about the science behind confidence is

how our bodies actually change when we feel truly secure in ourselves.

Our posture naturally improves, our breathing deepens, and our stress hormones decrease. Through EFT, we're essentially teaching our nervous system that it's safe to shine.

Radiating Confidence

Take a gentle breath and feel your inner power. Notice the strength that radiates from your core. Let your body settle into this natural confidence.

Karate Chop Point
"I embody natural confidence..."
"My power flows freely..."
"I shine with authentic strength..."

Round 1

Side of Hand: "I wonder how this confidence feels..."
Eyebrow Point: "I notice my inner strength..."
Side of Eye: "I'm curious about my authority..."
Under Eye: "I explore this natural power..."
Under Nose: "I sense my authentic voice..."
Chin: "I feel this leadership quality..."
Collarbone: "I observe this quiet power..."
Under Arm: "I notice my creative force..."
Top of Head: "I discover my true presence..."

Round 2:

Side of Hand: "I stand in my power."

Eyebrow Point: "I express myself boldly."

Side of Eye: "I own my natural authority."

Under Eye: "I move through life assured."

Under Nose: "I speak with conviction."

Chin: "I embrace my natural leadership."

Collarbone: "I radiate quiet power."

Under Arm: "I create from strength."

Top of Head: "My confidence radiates outward."

Take a gentle breath and notice:

- Where do you feel this natural power?
- How has your confidence expanded?
- What new sense of authority is emerging?

Quick Emergency Version (for moments of doubt)

Focus on these points while taking slow breaths:

1. Collarbone: "I radiate confidence"
2. Under eye: "My power flows freely"
3. Top of head: "I stand strong"

Evening Reflection: Notice the moments today when confidence flowed naturally. What helped you find that power?

How did it feel to move through your day with complete authority?

Journey Check-In

You're entering the final days of your 21-day journey. Take a moment to reflect on how far you've come. What shifts have you noticed? Which sequences resonate most deeply?

Remember, this practice builds upon itself - each day adds another layer of peace to your foundation. You're doing beautiful work.

If you haven't yet, now's a great time to check out my YouTube channel to listen to these sequences as you tap!

Chapter 24

Day 19: Setting Boundaries

Our nervous systems are designed with an intrinsic sense of personal space - it's why we instinctively step back when someone stands too close.

But many of us have learned to override these natural protective signals, leading to anxiety and overwhelm.

The fascinating thing about Tapping is how it helps restore our body's natural ability to sense and protect its own limits.

When we tap while focusing on boundaries, we're actually strengthening the neural pathways that connect our instinctive boundary signals with conscious awareness.

Science shows that people with clear boundaries have lower cortisol levels and stronger immune systems - our bodies literally function better when we honor our limits. Unfortunately, I've learned this the hard way many times...

. . .

Creating Clear Boundaries

Take a gentle breath and feel the space that belongs to you. Notice the clear edges of your energy field. Let your body settle into this natural sovereignty.

Karate Chop Point

"I set healthy boundaries..."
"My limits protect me..."
"I honor my needs completely..."

Round 1
Side of Hand: "I'm curious about setting boundaries..."
Eyebrow Point: "I notice my need for space..."
Side of Eye: "I explore what feels right..."
Under Eye: "I sense my natural limits..."
Under Nose: "I observe my yes and no..."
Chin: "I feel my inner wisdom..."
Collarbone: "I discover my peaceful boundaries..."
Under Arm: "I notice when I need space..."
Top of Head: "I explore what serves me..."

Round 2
Side of Hand: "My boundaries bring freedom."
Eyebrow Point: "I communicate my limits clearly."
Side of Eye: "I maintain strong boundaries."
Under Eye: "I honor my energy."
Under Nose: "I say yes and no with ease."
Chin: "I trust my inner guidance."
Collarbone: "I protect my peace naturally."
Under Arm: "I create healthy space."
Top of Head: "My choices serve me well."

. . .

Take a gentle breath and notice:

- Where do you feel this natural protection?
- How has your relationship with boundaries shifted?
- What new sense of freedom is emerging?

Quick Emergency Version (for boundary-pushing moments)

Focus on these points while taking slow breaths:

1. Collarbone: "I maintain clear limits"
2. Under eye: "I protect my peace"
3. Top of head: "My space is sacred"

Evening Reflection: Notice the moments today when boundaries felt natural. What helped you find that clarity? How did it feel to honor your needs completely?

Chapter 25
Day 20: Finding Peace

The neuroscience of peace is fascinating - our brains are actually equipped with a natural tranquility network that can override our stress response.

When we consistently practice EFT, we're strengthening these neural pathways, making peace our brain's default setting rather than anxiety.

Research shows that regular mindfulness practices like tapping actually increase gray matter in areas of the brain associated with calm and well-being.

I've been amazed to witness how this transformation happens in my own nervous system.

What begins as moments of peace during tapping gradually expands into a deeper, more lasting serenity. It truly feels like we're teaching our bodies a new language - the language of tranquility - until it becomes our natural way of being.

Embodying Deep Peace

Take a gentle breath and feel the peace that lives within you. Notice the quiet strength at your core. Let your body settle into this natural serenity.

Karate Chop Point
"I embody perfect peace..."
"Tranquility flows through me..."
"I radiate natural calm..."

Round 1
Side of Hand: "I explore this peaceful feeling..."
Eyebrow Point: "I notice deep calm within..."
Side of Eye: "I sense this inner stillness..."
Under Eye: "I observe perfect peace..."
Under Nose: "I discover tranquil spaces..."
Chin: "I feel peace anchoring deeply..."
Collarbone: "I notice natural serenity..."
Under Arm: "I explore radiating peace..."
Top of Head: "I experience pure tranquility..."

Round 2
Side of Hand: "Peace fills my being."
Eyebrow Point: "I rest in deep peace."
Side of Eye: "I embrace inner stillness."
Under Eye: "I maintain perfect peace."
Under Nose: "I create peaceful spaces."
Chin: "I anchor deeply in peace."
Collarbone: "I embody natural calm."
Under Arm: "I radiate perfect peace."
Top of Head: "Serenity surrounds me."

Take a gentle breath and notice:

- Where do you feel this natural peace?
- How has your relationship with tranquility deepened?
- What new sense of serenity is emerging?

Quick Emergency Version (for intense moments)

Focus on these points while taking slow breaths:

1. Collarbone: "I embody peace"
2. Under eye: "Tranquility fills me"
3. Top of head: "I am serenity"

Evening Reflection: Notice the moments today when peace flowed naturally. What helped you find that tranquility? How did it feel to embody perfect peace?

Chapter 26

Day 21: Maintaining Calm

Over these past 21 days, you've been creating new neural pathways through consistent tapping. You've literally been rewiring your brain's stress response system, teaching it to access calm more easily. What began as conscious practice is becoming your natural state.

Think of it like building a new highway in your brain. At first, finding peace took focused effort. But with each tapping session, you've strengthened these calm pathways.

Research shows that after about three weeks of consistent practice, new neural patterns begin to stabilize - exactly where you are now.

Sustaining Your Peace

Take a gentle breath and feel how naturally peace flows now. Notice how your body remembers this feeling more easily. Let yourself settle into this new way of being.

Karate Chop Point
"I maintain perfect peace..."
"Calm flows naturally..."
"I sustain tranquility easily..."

Round 1

Side of Hand: "I explore this deep peace..."
Eyebrow Point: "I notice my peaceful nature..."
Side of Eye: "I discover my calm choices..."
Under Eye: "I sense natural serenity..."
Under Nose: "I feel lasting tranquility..."
Chin: "I observe growing peace..."
Collarbone: "I notice inner harmony..."
Under Arm: "I explore perfect peace..."
Top of Head: "I experience deep calm..."

Round 2

Side of Hand: "Peace lives within me."
Eyebrow Point: "I navigate life peacefully."
Side of Eye: "I choose peace always."
Under Eye: "I sustain natural peace."
Under Nose: "I create lasting calm."
Chin: "I embody lasting serenity."
Collarbone: "I maintain inner harmony."
Under Arm: "I anchor in perfect peace."
Top of Head: "My calm deepens daily."

Take a gentle breath and notice:

- Where do you feel this sustainable peace?
- How has your relationship with calm transformed?
- What new sense of permanence is emerging?

Quick Emergency Version (for maintaining peace)

Focus on these points while taking slow breaths:

1. Collarbone: "I sustain peace"
2. Under eye: "My calm grows"
3. Top of head: "Peace flows always"

Final Reflection: As you complete this journey, notice how differently you feel from day one. What has shifted most profoundly? How will you continue nurturing this peace?

Remember - this practice is yours forever, ready whenever you need it.

Chapter 27

Sustaining Your Practice: Moving Forward With Peace

Congratulations on completing your 21-day journey. You've developed a powerful toolkit for maintaining peace and calm in your life.

What You've Accomplished:

- Created new neural pathways for peace
- Developed a personal tapping practice
- Built a library of sequences for specific situations
- Learned to tune into your body's natural wisdom
- Established a foundation of lasting calm

Your Ongoing Practice:

Remember that tapping is always available to you. Like any skill, it strengthens with use.

Maintaining Your Practice

- Start with 5 minutes each morning
- Create a dedicated tapping space
- Keep this book accessible
- Track your progress in a journal (Get your free EFT journal at angelashbrook.com)
- Share your experience with others

Common Situations for Tapping:

- Before important meetings
- While waiting in line
- Before you go to sleep
- When you wake up
- During breaks at work
- Before social events
- When making decisions

Creating Your Own Sequences

Yes, you can create your own Tapping sequences! While I started out following traditional methods, the way I was taught EFT tapping caused me even more anxiety than I already had.

If I had to repeat one more "even though" statement, my body was going to shut down. It was doing the opposite of what EFT Tapping is *supposed* to do.

Because of this, I worked diligently to create my own type of flow and sequences. You can do the same, just listen to your inner self.

1. Notice what you're feeling
2. Choose points that feel right
3. Use words that resonate
4. Trust your intuitive guidance
5. Adapt existing sequences

Signs of Progress:

- Feeling more centered naturally
- Responding rather than reacting
- Noticing triggers earlier
- Recovering more quickly
- Trusting yourself more deeply
- Finding peace more easily
- Sleeping more soundly
- Making decisions with clarity

When to Return to Specific Days:

- Day 1: When anxiety feels intense
- Day 2: For morning anxiety
- Day 3: For physical symptoms
- Day 4: When thoughts race
- Day 5: For future worries
- Day 6: Before social events
- Day 7: When needing self-trust
- Days 8-21: For specific situations

Building Long-Term Success:

- Practice regularly, not just in crisis
- Notice small shifts

- Celebrate progress
- Trust the process
- Keep what works for you
- Adapt what needs adjustment
- Share with others when moved
- Return to basics when needed

Creating a Daily Practice

Morning

- Brief centering sequence
- Set peaceful intentions
- Choose key points for the day

Throughout the Day

- Quick touch-ins during transitions
- Emergency sequences as needed
- Mindful moments with tapping

Evening

- Release the day's tension
- Celebrate moments of peace
- Set intentions for rest

Peace isn't a destination - it's a practice. Your relationship with tapping will evolve and deepen over time.

Trust that you have everything you need to maintain and deepen your calm.

Special Considerations:

- Travel: Pack this book or save key sequences
- Busy Days: Use quick emergency sequences
- High Stress: Return to basics
- Health Issues: Work with your healthcare providers
- Deep Trauma: Seek professional support

You may now find yourself:

- Naturally responding to stress differently
- Teaching others simple sequences
- Creating your own unique combinations
- Discovering new applications
- Deepening your self-trust
- Building lasting resilience

You've done beautiful work these past 21 days. You've built a foundation of peace that will continue to serve you. Trust in your practice, trust in your progress, and most importantly, trust in yourself.

May this practice continue to bring you peace, clarity, and joy.

You have everything you need within you. Tapping simply helps you access your natural state of calm and peace.

Chapter 28

Continuing Your EFT Journey

What you've learned in these 21 days is just the beginning. The beauty of EFT lies in its versatility - once you understand the basics of working with your nervous system through tapping, you can apply this technique to virtually any area of your life.

The key is this fundamental shift in approach: instead of fighting against what we don't want, we tap while exploring what's possible.

This subtle but powerful change in perspective - asking "What if?" and "I wonder..." - opens new neural pathways and creates lasting transformation.

Want to deepen your practice? Visit my YouTube channel (Angel Ashbrook) or my website (angelashbrook.com) where you'll find guided audio versions of each sequence from this book.

Hearing these sequences can add another dimension to your tapping practice, as our nervous systems naturally attune to the calm presence of another voice.

Your body is always listening, always learning, always ready to create new patterns. Each time you tap, you're building a new relationship with your own inner wisdom and capabilities.

Chapter 29

Bonus! When Anxiety Feels Overwhelming: A Deeper Sequence

Sometimes anxiety can feel particularly intense - perhaps your heart is racing, your thoughts are spinning, or your chest feels tight.

This sequence invites you to move through these sensations with gentleness and curiosity.

Find a comfortable space where you can be fully present. Place your hand on your heart and take a soft breath.

Karate Chop

"I wonder what peace would feel like in this moment..."

"What if my body could remember its natural state of calm..."

"I'm open to discovering a new way of being..."

Round 1

Side of Hand: "I notice these racing thoughts..."

Eyebrow Point: "I explore what lies beyond anxiety..."

Side of Eye: "I sense potential clarity..."

Under Eye: "I observe my breath's rhythm..."

Under Nose: "I feel each calming tap..."

Chin: "I discover new patterns..."

Collarbone: "I notice my heart rate..."

Under Arm: "I explore peaceful possibilities..."

Top of Head: "I welcome spaciousness..."

Round 2

Side of Hand: "My thoughts slow naturally."

Eyebrow Point: "My body finds balance."

Side of Eye: "I see situations clearly."

Under Eye: "Peace flows through me."

Under Nose: "My shoulders soften easily."

Chin: "I welcome this journey."

Collarbone: "Calm flows naturally."

Under Arm: "New patterns emerge."

Top of Head: "My mind finds space."

Return to any points that feel particularly soothing, and tap there while saying:

"I am open to deeper peace..."

"My body knows the way to calm..."

"Each breath brings more ease..."

Chapter 30

BONUS: 100 Tapping Statements

These statements can be used on any of the 9 EFT tapping points, at any time. I created a mix of curiosity-driven statements and empowering ones, because I feel that curiosity is the first step.

If you want to work through your anxiety more thoroughly, visit my website angelashbrook.com to get your free EFT tapping journal prompts!

PHYSICAL SENSATIONS OF CALM

1. "I wonder what deep peace feels like in my body..."
2. "My shoulders soften naturally..."
3. "Each breath brings a wave of relaxation..."
4. "My heartbeat finds its peaceful rhythm..."
5. "Tension melts like snow in sunshine..."
6. "My muscles remember how to rest..."

7. "What if ease could flow through every cell..."
8. "My hands become peaceful and steady..."
9. "A gentle warmth spreads through my body..."
10. "My feet connect with solid ground..."

MENTAL CLARITY

11. "My mind settles like still water..."
12. "Thoughts flow with easy grace..."
13. "What if clarity could emerge naturally..."
14. "I discover spaces between thoughts..."
15. "My mind creates room for peace..."
16. "Each moment brings new clarity..."
17. "Wisdom surfaces effortlessly..."
18. "My thoughts align with serenity..."
19. "Mental chatter softens into quiet..."
20. "Understanding comes naturally..."

HEART & EMOTIONAL PEACE

21. "My heart opens to tranquility..."
22. "What if peace could become my natural state..."
23. "Emotions flow like gentle streams..."
24. "I welcome this feeling of calm..."
25. "My heart knows perfect peace..."
26. "Each moment brings emotional balance..."
27. "I discover new depths of serenity..."
28. "Joy bubbles up naturally..."
29. "My feelings settle into harmony..."
30. "Inner peace radiates outward..."

CONNECTION TO NATURE

31. "I flow like a peaceful river..."
32. "My breath moves like ocean waves..."
33. "What if I could be steady as mountains..."
34. "I grow strong like ancient trees..."
35. "Peace surrounds me like morning mist..."
36. "My energy flows like sunlight..."
37. "Nature's rhythm guides my calm..."
38. "I settle like leaves after rain..."
39. "Serenity spreads like moonlight..."
40. "My roots grow deep into peace..."

INNER STRENGTH

41. "Power flows from my center..."
42. "I access my inner wisdom..."
43. "What if strength could feel peaceful..."
44. "My core radiates calm..."
45. "Each breath builds quiet confidence..."
46. "I discover my natural authority..."
47. "Peace and power flow together..."
48. "My inner light shines bright..."
49. "Strength emerges from stillness..."
50. "I embody a peaceful presence..."

TIME & PRESENCE

51. "This moment holds perfect peace..."
52. "Today I welcome peace..."
53. "What if every breath brought new calm..."
54. "I settle into the present moment with ease..."
55. "Time flows at the most aligned pace..."
56. "Each second brings fresh serenity..."
57. "I discover timeless tranquility..."
58. "Peace fills this endless moment..."
59. "Now is my peaceful sanctuary..."
60. "Present moment awareness soothes..."

ENERGY & FLOW

61. "Energy moves with aligned balance..."
62. "My vitality flows smoothly..."
63. "What if peace could pulse through me..."
64. "I discover my natural rhythm..."
65. "Each movement flows naturally..."
66. "Life force flows effortlessly..."
67. "I dance with peaceful energy..."
68. "Harmony courses through my veins..."
69. "My energy field expands gently..."
70. "Peace circulates freely..."

SAFE SPACES

71. "I create peaceful sanctuaries..."
72. "Safety surrounds me naturally..."
73. "What if everywhere felt peaceful..."
74. "My space holds perfect calm..."
75. "Each boundary brings more peace..."
76. "I discover new havens of rest..."
77. "Security flows from within..."
78. "My environment nurtures peace..."
79. "I belong in this tranquility..."
80. "Peace permeates my surroundings..."

GROWTH & TRANSFORMATION

81. "I bloom in peaceful ways..."
82. "Each day brings new serenity..."
83. "What if peace could keep expanding..."
84. "I discover endless calm..."
85. "Growth feels natural and easy..."
86. "Peace deepens like roots..."
87. "I evolve into deeper peace..."
88. "Tranquility grows stronger..."
89. "My calm presence ripples outward..."
90. "Serenity multiplies naturally..."

DIVINE CONNECTION

91. "Universal peace flows through me..."
92. "I connect with infinite calm..."
93. "What if divine peace surrounds me..."
94. "Wisdom guides me naturally..."
95. "Each breath connects me to calm..."
96. "I discover boundless serenity..."
97. "Peace transcends all limits..."
98. "Divine calm embraces me..."
99. "I rest in universal harmony..."
100. "Serenity becomes my natural state..."

Friend - I can call you friend, right? I mean, we just spent 21 days together... and grew so much! Thank you for your support in reading my book; it's greatly appreciated.

Please connect via my website and/or YouTube! I'd love to hear how these sequences have helped you, or what types of sequences you'd like me to create in the future.

Xoxo,

Angel